TREASURE

Gifts Received from
Challenges, Struggles, and Trauma

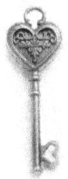

PAMELA STARUSTA

ISBN: (Paperback) 979-8-9917807-0-4
eISBN: 979-8-9917807-1-1

Table of Contents

Content Warning

This book contains writing that some may find disturbing, including incidents of emotional abuse, sexual abuse, physical abuse, and self-harm.

Introduction

This journey is deeply personal to me, but it is also universal. Whether your challenges mirror mine or are different, the principles of healing and self-discovery apply to all of us. Emotional scars leave their mark on us, shaping who we become, how we love, and what we do. I discovered that no matter how positive I tried to be, there was always a deep-seated fear and sadness lurking beneath the surface. This invisible force, though silent, was incredibly powerful, quietly shaping my life in ways I didn't fully understand. It was like an enemy within, robbing me of the joy of life—the real abuser, the real rapist.

I know what it feels like to be trapped in darkness. I also know what it feels like to rediscover the light within and the peace that comes with healing. This book is a guide to navigating the rough seas of life and finding your way back to the shores of healing, self-love, and self-discovery. I'm not a psychologist, psychiatrist, or social worker. What I offer comes from my own life experiences and the wisdom I've gained at The University of Life.

This story is not just one of survival—it's about thriving, reclaiming the parts of yourself that were lost, rediscovering your strength, and learning to live fully again. By the end of this book, my hope is that you will begin to see challenges, struggles, and trauma not as burdens but as gifts—gifts that will help you grow stronger, wiser, and more capable of living a fulfilling, happy life.

This personal transformation doesn't just benefit you; it has a profound impact on your loved ones, your relationships, your community, and society as a whole. Generation after generation inherit the unresolved pain and unhealed trauma of those who came before. You have the power, control, and the right to be the positive change that stops this cycle. As you heal, discover your goodness, and live happier and healthier lives, you change the world with the unstoppable ripple effect of healing.

As you read this book, know that you are not alone. I've been where you are, and I am here to guide you. Together, we will navigate the storms, uncover the treasures within, and find our way to a life filled with hope, strength, and happiness. This is your time to reclaim your joy, and I am honored to be a part of your journey.

Trauma to Triumph

"Someone I loved once gave me a box full of darkness. It took me years to understand that this too was a gift."

— *Mary Oliver*

My Personal Journey: A Prelude to Healing

I met my husband on my seventeenth birthday when my sister came home from Boston with a group of her college friends and threw me a surprise birthday party. He was one of those friends. At the time, I was recovering from anorexia. I was in what I call the chubby phase. Of course, nobody else thought I was chubby. It was the phase where my physical body no longer looked like a skeleton, but my emotional health was still recovering and vulnerable.

Fast forward thirty-five years to June 8, 2018. I woke up ready to face the day as always. I was fifty-two years old at the time. My husband and I had been together for thirty-five years and married for thirty. We had two beautiful boys. Our oldest son had graduated from college the previous month and was on his way to start his life and career in Chicago. Our youngest was a junior in high school. He said bye as he headed to work at the local Ace Hardware.

I continued with my morning routine: I went to Dunkin' Donuts, picked up two extra-large coffees and a bagel, and brought them home to have coffee time with my husband. We normally talked for an hour or so about the kids, and then he would segue into some version of how everybody and everything in his life had dealt him a raw deal. For the past few months he had been in a perpetual state of hate, and the conversations started and ended with nothing but hatred, anger, and negativity. I knew that the morning conversation would go just as it did. I knew what I had to do. I was to agree with any hatred or anger he expressed over coffee, or else I was guaranteed to have a terrible day. So, that is exactly what I did.

I made it through coffee time, agreeing, smiling, and adding the occasional "I know, right?" or "I can't believe it either" in response. Negativity and blame had become the daily mantra. *Whew, I made it through coffee time without saying the wrong thing.* The first goal of the day was accomplished.

Then, I could run some errands and be sure to return in a timely manner, and plan for the rest of the day. *Smile, be positive, agree. I've got this.* I had been living like that for three decades. *Watch what you say, or else everything could change. Remember, less is more. Show love. Don't say the wrong thing. Whatever you do, don't say the wrong thing.*

But for some reason, I said, "Hey, would it be okay with you if we stopped by my sister's house to drop off the graduation card for my nephew? It's only a couple of miles away. We can stay just a few minutes and come right back home. I hoped to get him his gift since he graduated three weeks ago."

The truth is, I know why I asked. I always wanted to see my family but wasn't allowed to. It was too risky; he needed to be in control. I knew I messed up. In my head, a voice said, *Pamela, why did you ask? You know better.* Only moments after I asked my question, I saw the expression on his face turn to complete rage.

We were standing in the foyer of our townhome. He violently kicked the inside of the front door, leaving behind a shoe print that went straight through the paint, exposing the metal below. Within seconds, I became the recipient of his built-up rage and anger. He grabbed me by the neck and slammed me against the wall, all the while screaming vile insults and spitting on my face to show me how worthless I was. He dragged me upstairs to our bedroom by my wrists. After about twenty minutes of repeated strikes to my body, choking, and spitting, I was forced onto my back with my husband's hand tightly holding my nose closed and my face being smothered with a pillow. He laid his six-foot tall, 230+ pound body on top of the pillow to ensure there was no room for air to get in. All the while, he was screaming, "I wish you were dead. I wish you were dead." As I was starting to fade away, I heard loud, repeated pounding noises. Suddenly, my husband was gone. I was breathing again.

Why am I here right now? I thought as the police officer was taking photographs of my wrists, arms, legs, and neck for his report. Less than thirty minutes ago, I was barely breathing. I was sitting at my kitchen table when the officer informed me that an anonymous person had called 911 and that my husband had been arrested. The state of Florida was pressing charges against him for domestic battery.

I told the police officer that my husband just got upset. I went on and on with excuses for why he was upset and tried to justify his behavior. The officer looked me straight in the eyes and said, "Do you know what you sound like to me?" I just stared back with a confused look, and the officer said, "An abused wife." I didn't respond, but in my head, I thought, *No, it can't be! I am not! This can't be true.* The officer handed me a pamphlet and told me to make an appointment with victim services at the Palm Beach County Courthouse as soon as possible.

A few days later, after my appointment at victim services, I was evaluated and diagnosed with PTSD. I received the results from the various tests and threat assessments, and everything was off the charts. I had to face the truth: I was an abused wife.

In the coming days and months, the floodgates of emotions and experiences came into my brain like a tidal wave held behind a retaining wall for thirty-five years. I felt like I was drowning in pain, shame, and fear. I had adapted to my environment, but now the walls were down. I needed those walls; they were my safety.

Somebody please help me. If this is freedom, I don't want it. I can't breathe, I can't hear, I can't think, and my ears are clogged. I can't survive like this, and I can't exist in my skin. I was trapped in a cycle of pain.

I was forced to face the cold, hard truth that I was the somebody that needed to help me. I hadn't taken any action to correct the situation; instead, I was only making excuses, lost in denial. I kept telling myself that my husband's behavior was just a result of stress or that he didn't really mean the hurtful things he said or did. I was holding onto the good moments in our life together. Those memories of laughter, love, and connection were like lifelines for me. I told myself that if we could just have more good times, everything would be okay. I convinced myself that things would eventually improve if I tried harder or loved him more.

Staying in that denial was one of the most difficult and damaging things I've ever done. By not taking action, I was allowing the abuse to continue and was contributing to my own suffering. I didn't want to admit that I was being mistreated or that my love was being used against me. I realize now that I was not only enabling his behavior but also diminishing my own worth. Coming to terms with this truth was painful but necessary.

Without delving further into the darkness, I want to tell you that I found a way to exist in my skin—I could, and I did.

According to the National Council for Mental Wellbeing 70 percent of US adults have experienced at least one traumatic event in their lives. I don't know the experiences you've had in your life or if you are one of the 223.4 million American adults who have suffered at least one traumatic event. What I do know is that if you have had past experiences that left you emotionally scarred, this book holds the promise of a transformative journey that can change your life.

I will share with you the wisdom I've gathered on my journey back to myself after years of abuse. This journey has been anything but easy; it has been filled with pain, fear, and countless moments of doubt. Yet, through all the darkness, I found light. I discovered that the path to healing is not just about overcoming the wounds inflicted by others but also about reclaiming the parts of us that were lost along the way. It's about rediscovering our strength, our worth, and our ability to love and be loved.

In the pages that follow, I will walk you through the lessons I've learned—not just as someone who survived, but as someone who has thrived despite the odds. This journey is deeply personal, but it is also universal. Whether you've faced similar challenges or different ones, the principles of healing and self-discovery apply to all of us.

We will explore the power of self-compassion, the importance of boundaries, and the necessity of confronting and embracing our pasts. I will provide you with practical tools and insights that you can use to navigate your own healing journey, no matter where you are starting from.

By the end of this book, I hope to help you see challenges, struggles, and trauma as gifts—something that, while painful, can be transformed into a source of strength and wisdom. This may seem impossible now, especially if you're still in the thick of your pain, but I assure you, it is possible. Through my own experience, I've come to understand that trauma does not define us—it refines us. It forces us to dig deep, discover parts of ourselves we didn't know existed, and emerge stronger, wiser, and more compassionate on the other side.

What's more, this transformation doesn't just benefit you. As you heal, your personal growth creates a wave of positivity and compassion that impacts the people around you in ways you can't even see. This ripple effect is one of the most beautiful aspects of the healing journey. It reaches your loved ones, friends, family, and extends outward exponentially, influencing even those you have never met.

This book is not just about surviving. It's about finding joy, peace, and purpose in a life that has been marked by trauma. It's about reclaiming your story, not as a victim, but as a warrior and a beacon of hope for others. As you read, I hope you will find the courage to embark on your journey of self-discovery and healing, knowing that you are not alone. I'm here with you, and together, we can turn pain into power, trauma into triumph, and wounds into wisdom.

In the chapters ahead, I will guide you across the open waters of discovery, understanding, and self-awareness. The destination? A land called the True Self. This new land is abundant with vibrant colors, beautiful sights, and the sounds of happiness. It's a place filled with limitless potential, where you'll find flowers named Self-Respect, Love, Courage, Gratitude, Joy, Kindness, Confidence, and so much more. The landscape is glowing with possibilities. As you explore, you'll discover the flowers you need to complete and empower yourself.

This land, where you will soon reside, is so peaceful and wonderful that most people think it only exists in their dreams. But I'm here to tell you it's real, and it won't take long to get there.

I'll show you the way. I've crossed this vast ocean before, faced the storms, and found the new land. Now, I'm here to share my map with you so you, too, can discover this beautiful destination. All the equipment you need to face the storms and navigate to this new land is already on your ship. Once you are ready and willing to pull up the anchor that holds you in port, you can begin your voyage.

When you finally set foot on this new land and feel the solid ground beneath you, breathe deeply, pause, and feel grateful for your safe arrival. After you've rested, you will embark on a quest for the treasure chest full of gifts and resources to help you flourish in this new world. The treasure map has been tucked away in your ship's cargo hold for decades. Now is the time to find it and dust it off. This map will lead you to the key and chest, and when you open it, you will uncover the riches needed to thrive in your new life.

When you're ready to pull up your anchor and set sail, turn the page.

Buried Alive

"Unexpressed emotions will never die. They are buried alive and will come forth later in uglier ways."

— Sigmund Freud

Welcome. I'm glad you decided to take this voyage. The first step in preparing for your journey to this wondrous new destination is to check your vessel and ensure all parts are in good working order. As captain of your ship, you are responsible for ensuring it is seaworthy. If any of your equipment needs repair, you must address it, or bring it to your crew's attention so they can assist you before setting sail.

I'm sharing this information with you because I wish I had done this earlier. It would have helped me avoid the shipwreck I ultimately found myself in. Let's start with the question of *Why?* Not "Why did he do this?" or "Why did this happen to me?" The real question is, "Why did I allow this in my life?"

I decided to grab some gear, go back in time, and take a deeper look at the condition of my vessel on my seventeenth birthday.

What I discovered was not good. I was not in tip-top shape. The truth is I would have been decommissioned and sent to the scrapyard if it hadn't been for my keel, which made up the foundation and stability of my ship, being in good condition. The rest of my vessel needed serious attention.

Much of the damage was below the surface, undetected by anyone. To see it, they would have needed to wear a wet suit, get a mask, an air tank, and some flippers, and take a deep dive.

Let's take a look at the parts of our vessel.

The **keel** is the main structural component of a ship that runs along its bottom, providing stability and strength. The keel represents the foundation of a person's life, the core values, beliefs, and inner strength that keep us grounded even in difficult times.

The **ballast system** of a ship ensures that it remains upright and stable, especially in rough waters. This draws a parallel to the mental and emotional balance we need in our lives.

The **cargo hold** of a ship is like your mind, where memories, experiences, and emotions are stored. Just as a ship must carefully manage its cargo to maintain balance and efficiency, we must be mindful of what we carry in our mental and emotional cargo holds.

The **propeller** of a ship is what drives it forward, creating the thrust necessary to move through the water. This is comparable to a person's motivation and passion—the internal forces that propel us toward our goals and dreams. We rely on our inner drive to push us forward in life and provide the momentum to overcome obstacles and continue moving toward our destinations.

The **rudder** is a small part of the ship compared to the rest but it plays a critical role in determining the vessel's direction. It's a powerful metaphor for our decision-making processes and the guidance we need to stay on course. In our lives, we need to have clear goals and the ability to make decisions that steer us toward where we truly want to go.

Finally, the ship's **wheel** and **anchor** represent our control over when and how we change direction or pause our journey. The wheel represents our ability to take charge and make conscious choices in our lives. Whether it's moving toward new opportunities or navigating away from danger, the wheel is our tool for changing the circumstances around us. Conversely, the anchor provides stability and security when we need to stop, rest, or hold our position. It's the part of us that knows when to pause, reflect, and regain our strength before continuing our journey.

What happens if any of these mechanisms are not working correctly? What happens if we leave for our voyage of life with damage to one or more of our systems? It would be dangerous, and we would likely get blown off course, diverted by unexpected storms; we could get lost, and possibly even shipwrecked. We could end up in a destination we had not intended to go to.

We could have set out on this voyage of life with a destination in mind but come upon a storm or bad weather and ended up anchoring in an unintended destination.

If your ship has been damaged for any reason, it is your responsibility as captain to assess the status or rely on your crew to diagnose the problem. You may even need to return to port and have a specialist address any issues outside of your skill set.

If the captain has an ineffective response to the operational failures on their vessel, ignores them, and sets sail anyway, it is doubtful they will make it to the destination, and it will be a rough ride.

When my vessel was created, it came out of production, shining and bright. It was destined for love, joy, kindness, and a beautiful life. My ship had a wonderful, loving crew that kept me in pristine condition. But what I failed to address was that my ship encountered a storm thirteen years after it was created, causing tremendous damage and blowing my voyage off course for forty years, ultimately leading to a shipwreck.

I had just finished seventh grade and was excited to start summer break with thoughts of sun, fun, and friends. My mother was a stay-at-home mom, and we were always allowed to have our friends over to hang out, live life, and enjoy what childhood was meant to be. But on this day, things were different. My mother was going to see a Broadway show in New York City. We were thrilled for her and couldn't wait to hear how amazing the show was when she returned home that evening. My mother always had a way of making every story magical and full of life. I couldn't wait to hear all about it. *Dinner time is going to be amazing tonight,* I thought to myself. *I can't wait.*

It was summer break, and we all had lots of free time. I invited my boyfriend over in the afternoon. We sat on the dark brown, plaid couch in the family room, sneaking kisses. If we heard my sister or brother coming, we would stop. I'm sure my blushing cheeks would give away the mischief I was involved in, but I didn't care. I had butterflies. I felt so special; *I'm in love,* I thought. *I'm in love.* What a wonderful feeling. I couldn't have been happier at that moment.

My brother went to play baseball with neighborhood friends outside, and my sister said, "Hey, Pammy, I'm going for a quick bike ride. I'll be back."

"Have fun," I said in return.

Within moments of my sister closing the door behind her, my boyfriend turned to me and said, "Hey, your mom's not home. Let's go upstairs to your room."

"I really don't think we should. You know, house rules, no boyfriends upstairs," I replied.

"Your mom's not here. Who will know? Come on, don't be so boring," he added.

I was filling up with guilt, but I thought, *I'm not boring.*

We lay down on the twin bed in my bedroom, and we kissed. I was overflowing with feelings of excitement. I felt like I had a roost of butterflies in my stomach. It was risky enough to kiss downstairs on the couch, but to lie down and kiss, now, this was exhilarating. *I hope I feel this way forever,* I thought to myself. *This is the best day of my life. So exciting, so beautiful.* The joy of adolescence and innocent discovery. The only way to describe this moment is it was pure joy.

Suddenly, the skies became dark, and the beautiful butterflies dancing in my stomach, creating feelings of elation and joy, flew away, leaving me empty inside. The weather was about to change; a storm had arrived. This wasn't the best day of my life after all.

I lay curled up on my bed when the storm had passed, feeling seasick. A part of my body below my waist and above my thighs felt sore. There were droplets of blood on my white bedspread. I was broken and damaged from the inside out. My virginity was taken without my consent, and I was left with just a shell of myself.

As I lay there sobbing, I thought, *Oh my gosh, my mom will be home within hours. What would I say? I am ashamed I can't admit this. I can't face this. I won't share this information with anyone. I'll keep it a secret. No one needs to know.*

I desperately scrubbed the evidence from my white bedspread until it looked like nothing had happened. Then, I took a shower, scrubbing my body with the same energy, though I was careful around the parts that were still sore. I combed my hair, put on fresh clothes, and finally forced a smile onto my face—a mask to complete the facade.

At dinner, I sat with my family, smiling and nodding along as my mother vividly recounted her magical experience at the Broadway show. It was filled with excitement, beauty, and joy. In our house, we focused on positive things, and this habit had been a big part of the happiness I had always known as a child. We all smiled and laughed, and I made sure to keep that smile on my face the entire time, even as my mind was miles away.

I managed to keep up the act. Throughout dinner, I forced myself to swallow the food that felt like stones in my stomach. I kept repeating to myself, *You can do this.* The alternative—facing the reality of what had happened—was unthinkable. I couldn't bear the thought of being the one to shatter the happiness of our family with this dark news. I felt responsible. After all, I allowed him upstairs. I broke the rules. I felt burdened with guilt and shame. I couldn't be the one to bring darkness and shame into our family. And I wouldn't.

Rape is the most under-reported crime; 63 percent of sexual assaults are not reported to police. Only 12 percent of child sexual abuse is reported to the authorities.[1]

Every day, I woke up and put on my mask, carefully crafting a smile that I wore like armor. It was my shield, the barrier between the world and the chaos inside me. No one could see the cracks, the shame gnawing at me like a hidden wound. But underneath it all, I was just trying to survive, desperately clinging to a sense of normalcy while hiding the scars that told a different story. The shame was like a shadow that followed me everywhere. I told myself that as long as I could keep up the facade and keep smiling, I could convince everyone, including myself, that I was okay.

I went through the motions—going to school, chatting with friends, acting as if everything was fine, and yes, continuing to date that same boyfriend. He told me, "If you break up with me, I'm going to tell everybody we had sex." I was horrified. His version of the story was different from mine. Of course, he blamed me for leading him on by taking him upstairs to my bedroom. When I asked him why he didn't stop when I was crying, screaming, and trying to push him off me, he dismissed it, claiming he knew I was just nervous and that deep down, I wanted him to do it.

Eventually, life moved on. I buried the pain, and I thought I was okay. The relationship was unhealthy, but I adjusted and adapted. I no longer felt the need to force a smile or pretend—until a year later, when he cheated on me and broke up with me. Six months after that, his stepdad was transferred out of state, and he was

---

[1] © National Sexual Violence Resource Center 2012, 2013, 2015. Nsvrc.org.

gone. That's when I learned the hard way that buried pain doesn't stay buried forever.

I was devastated. In my eyes, I had dedicated my life to him. I did everything he asked, and then he discarded me, leaving me feeling broken all over again. I was left with a sense of emptiness, and the unresolved emotional pain began to surface in unexpected and physical ways.

At fifteen years old, I woke up one morning feeling deeply emotional and overwhelmed with sadness. If anyone so much as looked at me, I felt like I was going to cry. I called my mom and asked her to pick me up from school, which she did. That night, I went to bed early, crying myself to sleep. The next morning, I woke up to find that the left side of my face was completely paralyzed. My lip was drawn downward, and I looked like I had suffered a stroke. My left eye wouldn't blink, and my eyelid stayed open.

My mother took me to the doctor immediately, where I was diagnosed with Ramsay Hunt syndrome. The doctors told me it was caused by an infection in my ear, but I know now that it was the built-up and buried emotional pain that had finally surfaced when I was discarded like worthless trash. The trauma I had buried for so long manifested physically as Ramsay Hunt syndrome.

Ramsay Hunt syndrome, similar to Bell's palsy, is caused by the herpes zoster virus. The factors that increase the risk of herpes zoster—stress, infection, malnutrition—were all present in my life. I was stressed, dealing with a flood of buried emotions that had resurfaced, and I wasn't prepared to handle the overwhelming pain, shame, and fear. Though I was given antiviral medication immediately, it took more than six months before I could begin to smile again. I went through electrical stimulation therapy and physical therapy, but even now, I still bear the lasting effects. Life became miserable again, but my crew never knew. I kept putting one foot in front of the other. I wasn't ready to face reality. I was embarrassed and ashamed.

I felt insecure going to high school with a paralyzed face and couldn't wait for summer break to arrive. When it finally came, I was relieved to stay in the safety of my home.

Reflecting on that period of my life, I realize that I had fallen into a victim mindset that stripped away my self-confidence and power. I did not take action; instead, I let fear of embarrassment and shame control my decisions. I needed to think logically, but I was unable to do so. I should have told a trusted person, someone who could help. But instead, I let external forces dictate the direction of my life. Limiting beliefs and emotional pain can hold us back, but recognizing and breaking free from them are essential for growth. Embracing discomfort and taking intentional, daily actions toward the true self allows you to navigate life's challenges and reach your full potential.

My experience with emotional trauma and its physical consequences taught me the importance of addressing emotional pain. Suppressing it only causes it to manifest in harmful ways. To maintain overall well-being, it's crucial to confront and heal from the emotional wounds that burden us.

Out of Balance

"What you resist, persists."

— Carl Jung

I made it through my freshman year of high school and was happy that summertime had finally arrived. For the first day or two of summer break I felt relieved. I could stay in the safety of my own home. The truth was that all these feelings, emotions, and fears that had surfaced were staying with me. It *wasn't* going to be the perfect summer vacation.

The distractions of school and life were helpful, but now those were gone, and it was just me, myself, and my thoughts and feelings.

I went upstairs to my bedroom, lay down on my twin bed, and allowed thoughts of self-hatred, shame, and embarrassment to run wild in my mind. I was cheated on, lied to, and discarded. I could not believe I was so stupid to think he cared about me. I honored him, was loyal, and did everything he asked, even after that painful summer day.

I leaned over to the nightstand and picked up the razor blade I had purposely placed there earlier that day. The blade was the double-edged kind that was sharp on both sides. The type of blade put inside one of those old-school razors a barber would use.

As I lay there looking at the shining light reflecting off the razor, I wondered about several things, including why I should even exist. *How and why do I want to live anymore?* Sitting there in the quiet, the weight of everything pressing down on me, I felt like I was drowning in my own thoughts. The pain, the exhaustion, it was all too much, and I couldn't see a way out. I kept thinking, *What's the point?* My world felt so cold and empty, and I was tired of pretending to be okay when every breath felt like a struggle. I thought about how easy it would be to just let go, to stop fighting, and finally find some peace. The idea of ending it all seemed like a release, a way to escape the relentless ache that had taken over my life. It felt like the only solution, the only way to make everything stop.

After these questions repeated through my head for several minutes and tears ran down my face, I sat up with my legs criss-crossed. I took a deep breath and felt calm inside for the first time in months. There were no sounds or smells; it was like I was in a vacuum. It was like floating in a sensory deprivation tank, quiet and serene. I enjoyed this peaceful feeling for what felt like an hour. Then, my thoughts of self-hatred, shame, and disappointment returned.

I thought about the people who might miss me, the things I'd never experience, and the impact my decision could have. It hit me that maybe, just maybe, there was still hope, still a chance for things to get better. The darkest cloud with all the lightning and thunder had passed over my room.

A smaller, grey cloud followed and hovered over my bed. This cloud was relaxing. It reminded me of the cozy feeling you get when you snuggle up on the couch under a blanket when the sky is dark and grey.

I calmly took the razor and cut across my knuckles slowly and repeatedly until droplets of blood landed on my white bedspread. As the sharp razor cut into my skin, it felt like a breath of fresh air. My emotional pain, sadness, and stress were replaced with the stinging sensation of pain. It was glorious.

Whenever the emotional pain became overwhelming, I would revisit my mental vacation spot, making sure to keep the results of my relaxation hidden. It was summertime, and bathing suits and shorts were my daily attire. It wasn't something I was proud of, but it was the only way I knew to make the emotional torment more tangible, something I could see and understand. It was a distraction from the unbearable thoughts swirling in my mind, a way to silence the noise, even if just for a little while. Each cut, each mark, was evidence of the pain I carried inside, a way to express what I couldn't put into words. The cycle of pain continued.

As much as it felt like an escape, I knew it was only a temporary fix, a Band-Aid on a wound festering beneath the surface. The relief was fleeting, and the guilt and shame that followed made the cycle harder to break. I was trapped in a pattern of hurting myself to numb the pain, but in doing so, I was only adding to the suffering. I wanted to stop and find a way to control myself, my thoughts, my body, something.

Within months of using self-inflicted harm (non-suicidal self-injury) as a coping mechanism, a new chapter of my life was about to begin. Welcome to the birth of the anorexia phase.

I learned that when we avoid confronting our emotional wounds, they don't simply fade into the background of our lives. Instead, these unresolved emotions linger beneath the surface, subtly influencing our thoughts, behaviors, and relationships. Like an untreated wound, these emotional injuries fester over time, becoming deeply embedded in our subconscious. While we might convince ourselves that we've moved past the pain, the truth is that these wounds continue to exist, often coloring our perceptions and responses in ways we don't even realize.

As time passes, unaddressed pain manifests in various aspects of our lives. It can show up as recurring patterns of unhealthy relationships, irrational fears, or persistent feelings of anxiety and depression. We might react disproportionately to certain situations, not because of what's happening in the present, but because old, unresolved emotions are being triggered. These resurfacing wounds can disrupt our lives, creating cycles of suffering that repeat until we confront the underlying issues. The more we ignore these emotional scars, the more they grow, affecting our well-being and our ability to live fully and authentically.

At sixteen years old, I became determined to take control of *something* in my life—my body. I said to myself, "I will take control of my body."

Every morning, the first thing I did was head straight to the bathroom. The scale was there, waiting for me like a judge, its cold surface a constant reminder of the battle I faced every single day. I would step on, holding my breath as if that could somehow change the number that appeared. When I saw it, my heart raced, whether the number was up or down by just a fraction of a pound. If it had gone down, I felt a fleeting sense of victory, a momentary high that told me I was still in control. But if it had gone up, even slightly, it felt as though the world was crumbling beneath me. My thoughts spiraled into panic, fear, and disgust. I promised myself, *Today, I will eat even less, push my body harder, do whatever it takes to see that number drop again tomorrow.*

Throughout the day, the number haunted me, dictating every decision I made. I avoided food as much as I could, picking at meals and making excuses to skip them altogether. My stomach growled, but I pushed the hunger away, telling myself that this was what strength looked like. Every time I walked by the bathroom, I was tempted to step on the scale again—just to check, just to see if I had managed to lose anything since the last time. It became an obsession, the constant need to measure myself, to see if I was any closer to the unattainable ideal I had set for myself. Even when I knew that weighing myself so often didn't make sense, I couldn't stop. It was as if the scale held my worth in those numbers, and without it, I didn't know who I was.

I started wearing baggy clothes and sweatshirts to conceal my "achievements." This went on for several months. My parents became increasingly concerned and tried to get me to eat more. Whenever they did, I would react irrationally—storming out of the house or shutting down and retreating to my room. It was a miserable time for my family.

One day, I weighed myself for the fifth time, taking off all my clothes before stepping onto the scale. In my haste, I forgot to lock the bathroom door. My sister opened it without knocking and saw my skeletal body standing on the scale, naked.

She screamed, "You look like a skeleton!" I jumped off the scale, placed my hand over her mouth, and quickly turned on the bathroom faucet, hoping to drown out her words. "Shhh, don't yell. Please stop yelling—Mom and Dad will hear you. Promise me, please, promise you won't say anything." She could see the utter fear in my eyes and promised not to tell. Only then could I breathe a sigh of relief.

But that night, unable to sleep, my sister broke her promise. She woke my parents in the middle of the night, pleading with them to get me help. By then, I was so frail that I occasionally fainted from normal activities like standing or walking up the stairs. Looking back, I'm thankful my sister and crewmate took action that day.

My parents sent me to therapy, followed by family therapy. I hated it, but I started eating again. I realize now that anorexia was not just a need for control—it was also a cry for help. I was finally allowing others to see on the outside what I had been holding inside for so many years.

Fear had been driving my decisions, controlling my life. I had let my hand off the wheel and no longer directed my vessel. I had lost my propeller, and with it, my power to move forward.

Based on statistics from the CDC in the National Intimate Partner and Sexual Violence Survey, 41 percent of women and 26 percent of men experienced contact sexual violence, physical violence, or stalking by an intimate partner during their lifetime and reported a related impact.[2]

---

[2] https://www.cdc.gov/intimate-partner-violence/about/index.html

These wounds might have healed had I confided in someone who truly cared. It's crucial to stand firm, voice your pain, and seek support when others wrong you. Never let fear silence your truth.

Looking back, I realize that much of my suffering could have been avoided if I had shared my experiences with someone who cared. I allowed fear to control my life, unaware that my past was dictating my future. Understanding the root cause of negative emotions or trauma is essential for living a happy and fulfilling life. Without identifying the underlying source of your pain, it becomes difficult to fully heal and move forward. Unresolved emotions often resurface, manifesting in unhealthy behaviors or thoughts that hinder well-being. By confronting and exploring these deep-seated issues, you too can break the cycle and begin to heal.

The path to healing emotional wounds requires acknowledging their existence and facing the pain they carry. It's only by bringing these hidden wounds into the light that we can start to heal them. This process may be difficult and uncomfortable, but it is essential for breaking free from the patterns that hold us back. By addressing our emotional injuries with compassion and seeking the help we need, we can transform our pain into growth, allowing us to move forward with greater clarity, peace, and resilience. Healing these wounds not only restores our emotional balance but also empowers us to live a life no longer dictated by the shadows of our past. Gaining clarity and releasing the shadows' hold can create a path toward genuine healing. This self-awareness not only empowers you to break free from the past, but also opens the door to lasting happiness and a more fulfilling life.

Looking back, I realized I hadn't acknowledged my emotional wound. Instead, I cultivated an adaptability mindset, which became my identity's foundation. These traits guided me through an abusive marriage that spanned over three decades, shaping much of my life. I found myself off course, still haunted by the emotional scars of my past.

Break the Bondage of Fear

"Indecision is the seedling of fear."

— Napoleon Hill

When I started therapy at victim services in the summer of 2018, I was fifty-two years old. I was overwhelmed with fear. The trauma of recent events had left me battling with PTSD, and I was struggling to find a sense of normalcy in my life. Therapy became a space where I could start to unpack my past and understand its impact on my present. We delved into the changes I needed to make to move forward, focusing on self-acceptance and understanding the behaviors that had emerged as coping mechanisms. This process was challenging but necessary for my recovery.

At the time of my husband's arrest, I was running my own real estate brokerage. The rapid changes in my life, combined with the emotional turmoil, triggered a severe onset of PTSD. Simple activities like going outside or driving became sources of intense fear. The situation was made worse by the fact that even after his arrest, my husband continued to stalk me, reinforcing my fears and making it nearly impossible to feel safe. The constant dread of his presence was suffocating, and the external factors beyond my control only intensified my anxiety.

In an effort to survive, I found myself retreating inward. The fear and anxiety isolated me from the world, leaving me lonely and desperate for a sense of control. Cleaning the house became my refuge—something I could manage when everything else felt over-whelming. The act of cleaning, though mundane, provided a small semblance of order in a life that had been thrown into chaos. Yet, despite this, the underlying anxiety and fear continued to domi-nate my days.

Walking the dog in the backyard felt like the safest option, given the high walls that enclosed the space. Although the open areas to the left and right were visible, the security of the yard provided a sense of comfort. However, when my parents visited, they took extra measures to fortify my home. They installed new locks and cameras, adding layers of security that made me feel more protected. Afterward, they took me to my sister's house for dinner, offering a brief reprieve from the tension that had been building.

When we returned home that evening, I decided to take the dog for a walk out front. My dad followed a few feet behind me as night had already fallen. The darkness made every sound feel more significant, and as I walked, we heard a car engine start. To our shock, we watched as my husband, attempting to conceal himself, leaned back in his seat, trying to hide between the driver's door and the passenger door of a charcoal-gray Corolla. The sight left us uneasy, adding to the complex emotions and fears that had been lingering in the background.

The day after the incident, I went to victim services, determined to take action to protect myself. I requested and was granted an extended restraining order, which would remain in place until our July court date. The detectives attempted to serve my husband at his mother's house a few days later, but he wasn't there, leaving me still feeling vulnerable and unsafe. I needed him to be served with this extended restraining order. The temporary one was expiring in a few days, and I desperately needed any sense of security, but it continued to elude me.

A week later, I decided to confront my fear head-on by going outside to take my dachshund, Daisy, for a walk. I wanted to see if I could reclaim some sense of normalcy and safety in the world. However, as I ventured just forty yards from my house, I saw a charcoal-gray Corolla driving into my complex. My heart dropped as I recognized him through the windshield—it was my husband. Panic surged through me, and I ran back inside, immediately calling the police.

The police responded quickly. I provided them with a copy of the original restraining order. Their investigation led them to a hotel less than two miles from my house, where they found him staying, along with the charcoal-gray rental car. He was arrested and served with the restraining order, which would be in effect until our court date in July. Though the immediate threat was removed, the encounter left me shaken, reminding me just how fragile my sense of safety still was.

We had our day in court in July, and I was granted a two-year restraining order. The court made it clear that if my husband stalked me or attempted to make contact, he would be sent directly to jail without any further questions. After the hearing, they kept him inside the courtroom and held him for fifteen minutes to give me time to leave the courthouse safely. I left quickly, and as I stepped outside, my nephew and his wife were waiting with my youngest son in the car. They drove us straight to the airport, where my son and I left town for six weeks.

Those six weeks away were a much-needed escape. I used the time to feel safe, surrounded by love, and begin the process of healing. My mind was still confused, but the distance provided a space to grieve without the constant shadow of fear hanging over me. Being away allowed me to reflect on everything that had happened and start to make sense of my emotions. It was a period of recovery during which I could focus on myself and begin to mend the deep wounds that had been inflicted.

During that time, I reconnected with my family in a way I hadn't in over thirty years. They welcomed me back with open arms and unconditional love, something I hadn't realized how much I needed. They were shocked to learn about what I had been going through, especially since I had never shared any of it with them before. My family had always thought it was strange that we rarely spent time together, but they had no idea the situation was this dire. For the first time in decades, I felt truly supported, and it made all the difference in beginning to heal.

When my family asked why I had never spoken about the abuse, I found myself questioning it as well. Why had I kept it all inside for so long? As I searched for answers, I traced it back to a single night when I was twenty-four years old. At that time, my parents and I weren't speaking, and they lived over a thousand miles away. It suddenly dawned on me that our estrangement had been the result of manipulation orchestrated by my husband. He had carefully engineered the rift between us as part of his plan to isolate and control me, and unfortunately, it had worked.

That particular night stands out as the worst of my life. We were dog-sitting for a friend, and the distance between the houses was just enough that no one could hear what was about to happen. My husband became enraged for no specific reason other than his need to release his anger. The violence and torture that ensued was terrifying. I kept thinking, *I am human, I am human, I know I am human.*

The abuse lasted for hours. It was in the early morning hours, and I was exhausted. My eyes kept closing. I did not want them to, but my eyelids felt so heavy. He would slap me and splash water in my face to keep me awake. He was frustrated with my lack of attention to his need for me to be alert. He thought it meant I didn't care for him or love him.

He went to the closet and grabbed a loaded gun. He flashed it around my face, yelling threats and insults. He stood behind me, wrapped his arm around my neck firmly, and placed the cold barrel of the gun on my temple. "Do you want to die tonight?" he screamed in my ear, spitting on my face. I stayed quiet. I was numb. My first thought was, *Why not?*

I felt calm at that moment. I was no longer spending my energy and thoughts on how to stop the pain, and my mind was at peace. I could think clearly for the first time that evening. I thought to myself, *If I don't die tonight, I'm leaving him.*

Eventually, he tired, and I waited anxiously for him to fall asleep. As soon as I was sure he was sleeping, I quietly slipped out of the house with nothing but the clothes on my back. It was 4:00 a.m. by the time I made my escape. With nowhere else to go, I headed to a local hotel. I felt completely isolated, with no family to call since we weren't speaking at the time. Looking back, I realize they would have accepted my call, but at that moment, I was in such a state of emotional confusion that I couldn't think clearly. I wouldn't have even known what to say to them.

In my disoriented state, I decided to call a friend who was also my neighbor. I didn't share any details about the abuse, only that my husband and I had had a fight. The reason I reached out to her was simple—I needed someone to know where I was. The real reason was to feel like I still existed as a human being. I told her I was at the hotel and needed time to think, asking her to check on me the next day. I promised to update her with more details later, but at that moment, I just needed reassurance that someone knew I existed, even if only temporarily.

I was sore and emotionally depleted. I wasn't thinking straight. I had no money and no one to go to. *Should I get in the car and drive? Just drive and not look back? But where would I go? Would I just be hiding for the rest of my life?* All these thoughts were so scary, and I didn't know what to do.

I turned on the shower, allowed the water to heat up, and stepped in. It was a moment of freedom, and I was overflowing with appreciation for the relaxation provided by the warmth of the water and the smell of the soap. I felt like I was experiencing life's pleasures through a magnifying glass. It was wondrous. I could feel every nerve ending on my skin tingle as I slid the washcloth across my arms, neck, and back.

I took a deep breath and was grateful for the joy of this moment. I added more soap to the washcloth, inhaled slowly , and enjoyed the smell of lemon and ginger. It was vibrant and refreshing. I reached down to clean the bottom of my torso. I raised my hand to rinse and repeat, and I was jolted from this joyous moment by the sight of rose-colored water running down my arm and chest as the water flowed through the washcloth. I thought to myself, *I need some sleep.*

I was abruptly awakened by the phone ringing in my hotel room. Fear surged through me as I hesitantly answered, only to hear the hotel clerk on the other end informing me that my credit card had declined. He said I needed to bring another form of payment, and I muttered an "okay" before hanging up. Panic set in as I realized I had no other means to pay. I began to worry—*How will I buy gas? Where will I live?* The uncertainty of my situation was overwhelming, and I felt utterly trapped.

A knock came at the door as I was lost in these anxious thoughts. Assuming it was the hotel clerk, I opened it, only to find my husband standing there. He had found me. The terror of that moment was paralyzing, and in that instant, I made a decision that would shape the years to come. I resolved never to share any information with anyone again.

Though I realize now that this was the wrong choice, at the time it felt like the only way to survive. Instead of seeking help, I chose to adapt and endure in silence, hiding the abuse from everyone around me.

Mayday! Mayday! Mayday! My Vessel Is Shipwrecked

For the next three decades, I remained confined within the walls of my vessel, channeling all my energy into adapting, learning, and surviving within the environment that had been shaped by years of fear and control. In a way, I found a strange comfort in this routine, as it allowed me to focus solely on survival without the burden of hope or dreams. I no longer wished for or envisioned a better life; instead, I accepted the reality I was living in, believing that enduring it was the best I could do.

Reflecting on that period of my life, I can see now how deeply entrenched I was in a victim mindset. I didn't realize it at the time, but I had completely internalized the belief that I was powerless, that my life was dictated by circumstances beyond my control. Every day, I woke up feeling as though I was at the mercy of everything and everyone around me. I convinced myself that I had no choice but to endure the pain, the fear, and the shame because that was just my reality. I was constantly on edge, always bracing for the next outburst, whether it was physical or emotional. I believed that the only way to survive was to adapt, and to hide behind a facade that told the world I was fine when, in truth, I was anything but.

I see now how that mindset robbed me of so much. It kept me trapped in a cycle of self-blame and self-doubt, where I believed that if I could just be better, or more understanding, then maybe things would change. But deep down, I knew that nothing I did could ever make it better, and that realization only fed into my sense of hopelessness. I stopped dreaming, stopped believing I deserved anything more than the life I was living. I became a passenger in my own life, allowing others to dictate the direction because I didn't believe I had the right or the strength to take the wheel. The thought of taking action, of standing up for myself, seemed impossible, as if the very idea of it was beyond my reach.

What I didn't understand back then was how much power I was giving away by clinging to that mindset. I let my fears and insecurities define me, shape my decisions, and limit my potential. I became so focused on what was being done to me that I lost sight of what I could do for myself. I didn't see the strength that was within me, the resilience that had kept me going all that time. Instead, I only saw my weaknesses, my failures, and the things I couldn't change. I let the victim narrative take over, and in doing so, I allowed it to dictate the terms of my life, making it harder to break free from the cycle of abuse and self-doubt.

When a child is born, they enter the world as a unique and beautiful being, brimming with limitless potential and an open mind. They are full of wonder, acceptance, and love, eager to explore the world around them. For many children, bedtime is a magical time filled with stories of enchanted forests, butterflies, and caterpillars—a world where imagination knows no bounds, and anything seems possible. In these early years, their minds are free to dream and discover, unburdened by the constraints of the world.

However, as we grow from early childhood into adulthood, this sense of limitless potential and wonder often fades. The boundless imagination of youth becomes overshadowed by the experiences, judgments, and limits imposed by society. Slowly, the innocence and openness of childhood are replaced by the weight of expectations and the opinions of others. We start to view the world through the lenses of those around us, adopting their fears, biases, and restrictions as our own, often without even realizing it.

As a result, many of us drift into a not-so-restful slumber each night, our minds filled with negative opinions, worries, and inherited fears. We carry with us the unhealed emotions and experiences of the people we are surrounded by, shaping our thoughts and limiting our potential. The magic and wonder of childhood seem distant, replaced by the complexities and anxieties of adult life. In this way, we lose touch with the limitless possibilities that once seemed so natural, forgetting that the world is still full of wonder if we only allow ourselves to see it.

If you find yourself in a perpetual state of stormy weather, think about your experiences and how they have shaped you as a person— your habits and your behaviors. Look further back than you think. That is where the answers live.

What if you could change your response to one event or experience in your past? What is the experience? How would you respond differently? How would your revised response have changed your life and the lives of the people around you?

If I could go back in time and change my response to a single experience in my life, I would go back to the summer storm. I would still lay curled up on my bed, feeling sick, broken, and damaged from the inside out. My virginity would still have been taken by force. I would still be left with a shell of myself, and I would have joined the family dinner, all the while choking down my food. What I would have done differently is to have spoken privately to my mother about what happened as soon as possible.

My whole life would have been very different. I was allowing fear to control my decisions, and the price I paid was far more costly than the tears my mother and I would have cried together instead of taking damage to my ship and ignoring it. As the captain of my ship, I was responsible for taking action.

I was wrong in thinking I was in control of my life by going along with the threats, adapting, and surviving. The truth is that from that moment forward, life was controlling me. My actions and behaviors were responses to external forces. I was steering directly into every storm in the open ocean. I couldn't imagine a new, beautiful land. I wasn't even searching for it because I focused on fear and trying to survive with the least amount of suffering. I created behaviors of adjusting and adapting to survive, not to live.

Now, take a moment and fast-forward five years into the future. Based on your behaviors and actions in your present life, is there anything you wish you would do differently? Do you think you will have regrets?

Is there an action, way of thinking, or behavior you believe you can or should change today?

Obviously, you can't go back in time, but you can make changes that will affect the rest of your life. It is your choice. It has always been your choice.

If your ship has been sailing lost at sea because of fears, beliefs, and catastrophic failures to address the root of the damage, it's time to change course.

It helped me when I was able to understand, on a scientific level, why these behaviors plagued my life. In the next chapter, I will give you the knowledge to understand, accept, and commit to facing new fears that come your way by understanding their origin and addressing them from a different perspective.

The Invisible Force

"Until you make the unconscious conscious, it will direct your life, and you will call it fate."

— Carl Jung

The conscious and subconscious minds are key players in shaping our thoughts, behaviors, and experiences. The conscious mind, the part of our awareness that we actively engage with, is where we make decisions, solve problems, and think logically. It's the part of our mind that allows us to navigate the world with intention, focusing on what is immediately before us. Though a small fraction of our mental processes, this conscious mind is the seat of our power, our ability to make choices and decisions.

Beneath the surface lies the subconscious mind, a vast and powerful invisible force influencing our beliefs, emotions, and behaviors, often without our awareness. The subconscious mind stores all our past experiences, memories, and learned behaviors. It is the seat of our automatic responses and ingrained habits, operating like a vast database that guides us based on what we have internalized over time.

While the conscious mind is active and deliberate, the subconscious mind is more passive, yet it has a profound impact on our lives. It can drive us to act in certain ways without us even realizing it, especially in situations that trigger deep-seated fears or anxieties. Trauma and negative experiences from the past are stored in our subconscious and later reveal themselves as irrational fears or phobias, influencing our actions and decisions.

The fears that arise from the subconscious are often not understood or controlled by the conscious mind. These fears usually stem from childhood experiences, societal conditioning, or unresolved emotional scars. Even if we consciously recognize that a fear is irrational, the subconscious mind can still exert its influence, making it difficult to overcome these fears. The language of the subconscious is emotions.

Understanding the interplay between the conscious and subconscious minds is not just interesting; it's crucial for personal growth and overcoming fears. By becoming aware of how the subconscious influences our lives, we can begin to address and reprogram the patterns that no longer serve us. Mindfulness, therapy, and self-reflection can help bring subconscious fears into conscious awareness, allowing us to confront and transform them. I have found in my experience that if you recognize the specific emotion that is attached to fear, you can consciously address, reduce, and, in many cases, eliminate the feeling of fear. This recognition is the first step toward empowerment and personal transformation.

Have you ever been at work, stressed, feeling like you will never finish all your work by the end of the day? Anxiety has set in; you're overwhelmed, and turmoil is stirring in your stomach. Now you have a tension headache, your muscles tighten, it's another stressful day at the office. The truth is you know you will not get fired, but you are responding with this overwhelming fear of failure anyway.

Most of us have experienced something similar in our lives. You can make it through the day, weeks, or years with relaxation techniques, deep breathing, and meditation. These are coping strategies that don't solve the problem. You will likely find yourself feeling the same way again and again. If something similar happens regularly in your life, you will benefit by searching deeper into your emotional fear. You are being driven by fear, but what exactly are you afraid of? Go deeper and discover the specific emotion to find the root cause.

You will likely be afraid that your coworkers or boss will see you as a loser, weak, or stupid. Ask yourself, "Why do I think I am a loser?" Or fill in the blanks. Did anyone or anything make you feel that way?

Go back to the first time you can recall feeling that specific emotion. Enter a no-judgment zone and be honest with yourself. Discovering the root cause of these fears and the **emotions attached** to them is crucial to clearing these blocks and ultimately living a happy and fulfilling life.

Fear is a valuable function of the subconscious that we are born with. The purpose is to protect us and keep us alive. We want to keep this natural fear.

The fears that we need to address are the ones that have been embedded in our subconscious by negative events, criticisms, and misguided views of people in our lives. These fears change us and drift us farther away from our true selves. They can wreak havoc on our lives and relationships, creating habits that do not serve us.

The good news is that once you become aware of the thoughts, emotions, and experiences that no longer serve you, you can address them and make a change. Cultivating a higher level of awareness is crucial. It allows us to consciously navigate our emotional landscape and make choices that align with our true desires and values.

We must take full responsibility for our emotional well-being to achieve inner peace and freedom. It's easy to fall into the trap of blaming others or external circumstances for how we feel or how our lives unfold, but this mindset only perpetuates a cycle of powerlessness.

True freedom comes when we realize that we can choose our responses to life's events. By taking ownership of our past, we empower ourselves to create the life we want rather than being victims of circumstance. This means acknowledging that our inner peace is our responsibility and that it's within our control to nurture and protect it.

I'm sure that through the stories I've shared with you about my life, it would be easy to want to blame my ex-boyfriend or ex-husband for all the emotional pain I endured. I understand if that is how you feel because that is exactly what I did for decades.

When someone violates you or shows you who they are, you must believe them. It's essential to ask yourself if the way you are being treated works for you, and if it doesn't, you need to make a choice and take action. I did not do that, and I paid a huge ransom for my own life. Inaction is still an action and a choice.

We can support, understand, and love others, but we cannot change them.

It's our responsibility to recognize our power and decide whether to stay or leave when mistreated. The choice is ours, and we must choose wisely because our life is on the line.

When I shifted my perspective, it was liberating. It allowed me to stop focusing on what my ex-boyfriend and ex-husband should have done differently and instead turn my attention to what I could have done to change the direction and experiences of my life.

It isn't about condoning their actions or denying the hurt they caused, but about reclaiming your power and taking responsibility for your own happiness.

It is not about making people or experiences the villains in my story but recognizing that, like all of us, they are struggling too. While compassion for the struggles and problems of other people is important, it doesn't diminish the need to prioritize my own well-being and take the steps necessary to build a life free from pain and fear.

Once I understood why I had made the choices I did in my past and accepted that I hadn't taken the necessary action, I was able to forgive myself. I was then able to forgive and release the negative emotions I harbored toward my ex-boyfriend and my ex-husband.

I've found peace in knowing that I reclaimed my power and made the choice to live a life that aligns with my values. It took me a long time to realize that it was never my responsibility to try and change or fix other people's problems.

I have gained knowledge and wisdom from my past and grown and evolved with a deeper understanding of life, people, and relationships. I left behind the pain.

Accepting your circumstances as they are—without resistance or denial—frees you from the mental and emotional turmoil that comes from wishing things were different. This acceptance doesn't mean complacency but rather a peaceful acknowledgment of the present, which allows you to channel your energy into creating the future you want.

Taking responsibility for your life also means being proactive about change. It's not enough to simply wish for a better life; you must take deliberate action to bring it into being. This involves focusing your energy and attention on your goals and being grateful for the opportunities that come your way.

Reveal Your Strength

"The weak can never forgive. Forgiveness is the attribute of the strong."

— Mahatma Gandhi

Achieving inner peace requires the practice of forgiveness, both toward others and yourself. It starts by identifying specific situations or relationships where you hold negative feelings. Reflect on how much power you give these external circumstances or people and how much you allow them to disrupt your inner peace. Recognize that by holding on to resentment, you are only harming yourself. Instead, practice self-forgiveness for any perceived shortcomings or fears fueling your resentment. Fully accept yourself and your past actions and make the conscious choice to let go of the negative emotions that are holding you back.

Forgiving those who have wronged you is essential to achieving inner peace. Understand that the hurtful actions of others often stem from *their* pain and choose to respond with compassion rather than resentment. This shift in perspective allows you to release these situations or people's hold on your emotional well-being. As you embrace forgiveness, you strengthen your inner peace, creating a space within yourself that cannot be shaken by external events or individuals. Remind yourself that your inner world is sacred and that only you have the power to protect it.

By practicing forgiveness, you reclaim your personal power. Your journey toward inner peace can serve as a powerful example to others, inspiring them to embrace forgiveness in their own lives. Use the calm and harmony you cultivate within yourself as a model to encourage more understanding and compassion in your life and relationships. Remember, the key lies in what is within your control—your thoughts, emotions, and actions. By focusing on these, you can transform your life and help create a ripple effect of peace and positivity in the world around you.

You may remember in the introduction of this book, I said that no matter how positive I tried to be, there was always a deep-seated fear or sadness lurking within me, silently shaping my life in ways I couldn't fully understand. This hidden force, though invisible, was incredibly powerful. It stole my time, happiness, and love and robbed me of joy. I didn't realize it then, but I hadn't truly forgiven myself or the cocreators of my past negative experiences. I thought my acceptance of the events that occurred was enough. It wasn't. I needed to accept, forgive, and release the negative emotion attached to the event. That is when I found true freedom.

Finding inner peace requires strength and courage, but I will say without a shadow of a doubt it is worth it 100 percent. For so long, the pain I felt consumed me, overshadowing any sense of peace. My path to healing began when I understood that forgiveness was not about excusing anyone else's behavior or diminishing the impact it had on my life; it was about freeing myself from the chains of shame and embarrassment that kept me tied to the past.

Forgiveness became an act of reclaiming my life, a conscious choice to no longer let the actions of others define me or my future. It didn't happen overnight, and it wasn't easy. There were days when the memories would resurface, and the pain would feel fresh again. But with each step, I learned to separate the person from the hurt, recognizing that forgiveness was more about my own healing than anyone else's. It was a way to release the past's grip on me and open space in my heart for peace and compassion—toward myself, most of all.

As I embraced forgiveness, I began to find a sense of inner peace that had eluded me for so long. It didn't mean forgetting about or dismissing what happened, but it allowed me to move forward without the weight of bitterness holding me back. Forgiving was a way of saying that I refused to let the pain define my life any longer. It was a declaration of my strength and resilience, a commitment to living a life rooted in peace rather than in the shadows of the past. In choosing forgiveness, I found the freedom to fully embrace the present and the courage to step into a future filled with hope and possibility. This moment was the breakthrough for me that made all the difference. All negative thoughts were gone. My focus was directed toward my future and not my past.

What we focus on is like a compass that guides our direction in life. Our thoughts and attention shape our actions, decisions, and our path. When we concentrate on what we want to achieve and the person we aspire to become, we align our efforts with those goals, steadily moving toward them. This focus acts as a powerful force, influencing our habits, attitudes, and daily choices, which collectively determine our success.

Moreover, by dedicating ourselves to personal growth and self-improvement, we strengthen our ability to navigate challenges and seize opportunities. Working harder on ourselves than anything else means investing in our skills, mindset, and well-being, ensuring that we constantly evolve and adapt. This continuous self-development not only enhances our capacity to reach our goals but also transforms us into the person we need to be to achieve them.

Gratitude is a powerful force and can shift your perspective, helping you see possibilities where others see obstacles. When you combine this proactive mindset with a deep sense of responsibility for your own happiness, you become the architect of your destiny, shaping a life that reflects your goals and values and your truest self.

Ultimately, the power to live a fulfilling and meaningful life lies within you. You align your life with your highest potential by elevating your consciousness, taking control of your inner peace, and focusing on what you truly want. This requires courage, self-awareness, and an unwavering commitment to your well-being. But as you embrace these principles, you'll find that life becomes richer, more purposeful, and deeply satisfying. Your happiness is your own to create, and with that power comes the freedom to live the life you've always imagined.

If you find that you are not living the life you want, it's likely that your perspective is your greatest limitation. A negative or limiting perspective can act as a prison, confining you to a life that falls short of your true potential. However, by shifting to a "power perspective," you open new possibilities. This power perspective is rooted in the belief that even if you don't know how to achieve your goals, you are committed to the journey and will find a way no matter what. This mindset turns obstacles into opportunities and failures into learning experiences. By embracing this perspective, you free yourself from the constraints of doubt and fear, allowing yourself to move forward with confidence and purpose.

All meaningful change begins from within. The first step toward transformation is being completely honest with yourself—acknowledging your current situation, recognizing your desires, and confronting the obstacles that have held you back. Without this self-awareness, it's impossible to chart a path forward. If you don't take the initiative to create a plan for your own life, you risk becoming a passenger in someone else's, fulfilling their goals rather than your own. This honesty is the foundation of personal growth; it's the moment when you stop living by default and start living by design.

Mastering your mind and attitude is the most crucial skill in this process of change. Your thoughts and beliefs shape your reality—how you perceive challenges, how you respond to setbacks, and how you pursue your goals. If you allow negative thoughts and self-doubt to dominate, you create a mental environment that limits your potential. This applies to all areas of your life.

On the other hand, by cultivating a positive and empowered mindset, you unlock the ability to overcome obstacles and achieve your aspirations. This mental mastery involves daily discipline, training your mind to focus on possibilities rather than limitations, and choosing resilience over defeat.

Ultimately, trusting your vision and taking consistent action are the keys to turning this internal change into external reality. Your vision and goals act as a compass, guiding your decisions and actions.

Trusting and believing in your ability to achieve them, even when the path ahead is unclear, is vital. It's about having faith in your resilience and resourcefulness. But vision alone is not enough; it must be coupled with action. No matter how small, every step you take brings you closer to your desired life. By continuously working on yourself, maintaining a positive attitude, and taking decisive action, you turn your dreams into reality, transforming your life from what it is to what it can be.

You now have the knowledge and wisdom needed to step onto the new land. Once you explore and discover the new land, living in this new environment will be your choice. Choose wisely. The choice you make will determine your future.

Reclaim Your Joy

"Life is like a sunrise; without a few clouds, you may not see its true beauty."

— *Pamela Starusta*

As you step onto this new land, the discovery of your true self begins.

When I arrived at this place in my life, I felt a profound sense of gratitude. Life appeared magnified in ways I had never expected. It was as if I had been given a second chance to see the world and myself with acceptance, appreciation, and love.

Every day felt like a precious gift, and I began to live with an overwhelming sense of joy and gratitude, savoring the small moments I once overlooked. I embraced the fullness of life, imperfections and all.

When the walls I had built around myself came down, my life became filled with joy and authenticity. With my newfound freedom, I could finally be the daughter, sister, mother, and friend I had always wanted to be.

For the first time in decades, I felt free to be myself, living in a world where each day was not just another day, but a bonus day—an opportunity to live, laugh, and love.

When I reconnected with my family, they all said the same thing: They couldn't believe I had resurfaced as the same person I was thirty years before. My dad said, "I finally got my beautiful, loving, kind daughter back. I thought we lost you forever." The memory of my dad making that statement still brings tears of joy to my eyes.

It is true. My true self was never lost. It felt like I was able to pick up right where my life had been diverted. I am thankful for that.

Now it is your time to step onto this new land; the discovery of your true self begins. I invite you to take my hand for the remainder of this chapter and allow me to walk beside you, guiding you through the experience of self-acceptance and the joyful vision of a positive and meaningful life. As you glimpse this possibility, remember it is your decision whether to take the steps to bring it to life. You hold the power, and I am here by your side, supporting you and cheering you on with love. When you are ready, read on.

You feel a sense of comfort over you, a feeling you haven't experienced in years. The serenity and peace of this place resonate with you as if you had been here before.

A warmth emanates from your heart, a feeling of love, compassion, and acceptance that fills your entire being. You are overflowing with emotions, and your heart feels warm and grateful. You breathe deeply, immerse yourself in this tranquil environment, exhale, and begin to explore and discover.

You take a few more steps and notice a large tree with a light shining on it up ahead. As you approach, you see a large mirror with a beautiful ornate frame. You look into the mirror and see the most beautiful person. You are deeply attracted to this person. You look past any flaws or imperfections and feel a deep sense of love, understanding, and compassion. Your heart feels warm and overflowing with gratitude and acceptance. You feel thankful, so very grateful, for this moment and this feeling.

You are curious to discover the amazing qualities that make this reflection uniquely beautiful. You notice the beautiful light shining as well as shadows from the tree. The combination of the bright light with the contrast of the shadows makes the image magnificent. Authentic, simply majestic. You feel a love growing inside you—of acceptance and the need to share the rest of your life with this imperfectly perfect reflection.

The feeling is intoxicating. It pulls you in. It feels safe and loving, without judgment—just acceptance and positivity. This person radiates a force that brings confidence, self-love, and inner peace. You know they are worthy of life's blessings and feel their love and kindness overflowing within you. You notice a few scars and frown lines, but in your heart, you feel these features magnify their beauty. They are beautiful, natural and picturesque, but not a picture. They are not a flat image that was taken by another. This person is authentic and real.

You reach into your back pocket and take out the treasure map that you retrieved from the cargo hold on your vessel. You dust it off, open it up, and start walking. You feel calm and ready. You forge ahead with a slow, consistent, and steady pace.

You come upon an open area. You see two clear paths—they look as though other people may have taken them before. The grass is worn, and you can see sections of soil from wear and tear. The map shows three paths, but you only see two. You step forward in the direction the map is leading you. You see a very small opening in the trees. The vegetation is dense, and there is tremendous over-growth, as if this path was abandoned decades ago.

You can envision the path, and you believe you have the strength, resilience, and resourcefulness to proceed. You have faith in your ability to navigate this abandoned path. You realize you may need to push beyond your limits, but you are excited and decide to move forward.

Early in your travels, you move slowly, cutting through heavy vines and weeds, continuing steadily. You know that every step you take, no matter how small, brings you closer to your destination. This time is different because it is for you.

You arrive at a waterfall and sit down on a large boulder, feeling the cool mist gently caress your face. The water cascades in a mes-merizing dance, its rhythmic roar both powerful and soothing. Around you, the lush greenery of the forest stands tall, vibrant with life. The trees, their leaves glistening with dew, form a natural canopy that filters the sunlight into soft, golden beams. The air is rich with the scent of damp earth and wildflowers, a fragrance that invigorates your senses and brings a deep sense of calm.

As you sit there, you notice the delicate interplay of nature. Tiny birds sit on the branches, their chirps adding their melody to the symphony of the waterfall. The smooth surface of the boulder beneath you is warm from the sun's rays, grounding you to the earth's energy. Nearby, a gentle breeze rustles the leaves. The moment feels timeless as if your life has paused to allow you to embrace this beautiful moment.

As you lay your head on a soft patch of moss growing between two rocks, you see a large key with a small scroll attached. You pick up the bronze key, open the scroll, and it reads *Si Vis Pacem, Para Bellum*. You are curious and eager to understand the meaning behind this discovery. You lay the bronze key on your chest directly over your heart and drift into a deep sleep.

As you dream, you find yourself in a place that seems to glow with an amazing light. You are in a beautiful village unlike anything you have ever seen. The air is fresh, the colors of the landscape are vibrant, and a sense of peace permeates everything around you. As you walk through the archway at the town entrance, you look up and see the inscription at the top of the arch: *Si Vis Pacem, Para Bellum. Just like the scroll*, you think to yourself.

You continue to explore this enchanting place, walking down a cobblestone street lined with quaint houses and gardens bursting with flowers. You see a person walking nearby and approach them.

"Excuse me." You ask, "Where am I, and if you don't mind me asking, what does the inscription on the arch mean?"

The person smiles warmly and replies, "You are in the beautiful world of your reality, and the saying is a Latin axiom that means, 'If you want peace, prepare for war.'"

Intrigued, you ask, "What makes this place so beautiful?"

With a gentle laugh, they respond, "Here, we all start each day with a deep sense of gratitude. We spend our days appreciating the beauty around us, and, most importantly, we accept and love ourselves fully. Self-love is the foundation of this place."

You notice there are no walls in the village. You mention this to the person, saying, "I notice that there are no walls here."

They nod and say, "We don't need walls. Fear has tried to come here, but it cannot survive because all of us are filled with inner peace and love. Love has power over fear. We treat each other with kindness and compassion. We are all very different, but the one thing that unites us is our respect and love for ourselves, each other, and the world we live in."

Standing there, you feel an overwhelming sense of peace and belonging. This village is a place where love and respect are not just ideals but the very fabric of life. It is a world where everyone values themselves and others, where the power of love creates a reality free from fear and judgment. As you take in the beauty of this magical place, you wonder if this dream is showing you a path to create a similar place in your waking life.

As you wake up, you reflect on your dream and the saying, *If you want peace, prepare for war,* and you realize how deeply it reso-nates with your journey toward personal well-being. You have come to understand that achieving inner peace isn't about avoid-ing challenges or pretending threats don't exist; it's about being prepared to face whatever challenges come your way. It is not just about physical safety but also about strengthening your heart and mind. You need to build resilience, set boundaries, and equip your-self with the tools to protect your emotional and mental health. By being ready to defend your peace—whether from external dangers or internal struggles—you can create a space where you feel safe, secure, and in control. This readiness is not a sign of fear but a declaration of your commitment to yourself, ensuring you are not caught off guard when life throws its inevitable challenges.

You open your eyes. As you sit up, the landscape around you slowly sharpens into focus, and there it is—a treasure chest right in front of you. For a moment, you stare at it, your mind trying to catch up with what your eyes are seeing. The chest is old, its wood dark and weathered, bound with iron that glistens in the light filtering through the trees. Your heart starts to beat faster with a mix of excitement and disbelief washing over you. You wonder how long it's been here, hidden away from the world, waiting for someone like you to find it. The thought sends a shiver down your spine. You reach out, your fingers brushing against the rough surface of the wood, feeling the grooves of the carvings that cover it, intricate patterns that seem to tell a story all their own.

You take a deep breath, preparing yourself for what comes next. You use the key to open the chest. As you carefully lift the treasure chest lid, the contents inside glimmer with mystery and significance. The first thing that catches your eye is a pile of radiant diamonds, their facets reflecting the light in a dazzling display of brilliance, symbolizing wealth and the value of inner strength. Beside them rests a bottle of olive oil, its golden glow representing nourishment and the essence of life.

Nestled next to the olive oil lies a bottle of red wine, symbolizing celebration, connection, and the joy found in shared experiences. Scattered among these treasures are an unlimited number of seeds, each one holding the promise of growth and new beginnings. The seeds signify that life can flourish when nurtured with care. Finally, you find a mirror, its polished surface inviting you to gaze upon your reflection. This mirror is more than just glass—it symbolizes self-awareness and the journey of self-discovery, reminding you that your greatest treasure lies within yourself.

You celebrate with a grateful smile for the discovery of this treasure. Your appreciation is magnified by the struggles you endured to arrive at this moment. You realize these gifts remind you what it took for you to get here.

The diamonds that are shining brightly as your treasure were created by *pressure*. The precious olive oil is extracted after the olives are *pressed*; the wine only exists after the grapes are *crushed*. The seeds *grow in darkness and light*. The mirror is vital for staying true to yourself always.

You pick up your treasure and walk until you find an open patch of land on the other side of a valley, where the landscape unfolds in a breathtaking panorama. As you stand there, you feel a deep sense of calm and fulfillment wash over you, as if the very landscape is welcoming you, embracing you in its serenity. The vastness of the open land makes you feel both small and limitless. It's a moment of pure connection between yourself and the world. All the worries and concerns that once weighed on you fade into the background. The beauty of this place, combined with the significance of what you've found, fills you with a quiet joy, a sense of purpose you haven't felt in a long time. With its open sky and endless horizon, this patch of land feels like the perfect place to reflect, breathe, and be.

You decide that instead of building walls made of bricks of pain, embarrassment, and shame that you thought kept you safe but really kept you isolated, lonely, and alone, this time will be different; you will surround your home with a large, vast beautiful flower bed that expands as far as your eyes can see. You will plant seeds from your treasure chest, nourish them with love, and watch them grow into the beautiful flowers that nature intended.

You will place a bench in the heart of your beautiful flower bed. This is no ordinary patch of flowers; it is a vibrant garden, carefully tended and cherished by nature itself. Each flower represents a different positive emotion, blooming in harmony to create a living tapestry of color and light.

At the center of the garden stands the **Lotus of Self-Love**, a resilient yet delicate flower. The lotus symbolizes purity and spiritual growth, blooming beautifully even in the murkiest waters. It represents the ability to rise above challenges and embrace oneself fully, reflecting the inner journey of self-acceptance and personal transformation.

Standing tall beside the lotus is the **Sunflower of Gratitude**, known for its ability to turn toward the sun, seeking the light. Sunflowers represent warmth, positivity, and appreciation, embodying the essence of gratitude as they stand tall and bright, always reaching for the good in life and reflecting a heart full of thankfulness.

Next to the sunflower, you see the **Rose of Self-Respect**. Its deep crimson petals radiate strength and dignity, reminding all who behold it of the importance of honoring oneself. The rose's sturdy stem symbolizes self-respect's inner foundation, allowing all other emotions to thrive around it.

Beside the rose grows the **Lily of Love**, pure and white, its delicate fragrance filling the air with warmth and compassion. The lily symbolizes the unconditional love that connects all living things, its petals unfolding like open arms, welcoming and embracing all who come near. With its gentle presence, this flower nourishes the entire garden, creating a bond that unifies the diverse blooms around it.

Nearby, the **Daisy of Forgiveness** sways gently in the breeze, its soft white petals tipped with a golden hue. The daisy represents the lightness that comes with letting go of past hurts. It whispers a reminder that forgiveness is the key to healing, its roots inter-twined with the earth, drawing strength from the wisdom that peace is found in release.

Standing tall beside the daisy is the **Carnation of Confidence**, a symbolic flower representing self-assurance, inner strength, and the unwavering belief in one's abilities. Its bold and vibrant petals reflect the certainty and poise that come with trusting oneself, serving as a reminder that true confidence blooms from within, radiating outward in every aspect of life.

The **Tulip of Courage** blossoms in a brilliant array of colors, sym-bolizing the bravery that arises from within. Its petals, though delicate, are solid and resilient, representing the courage needed to face the unknown. The tulip teaches the garden that true courage is not the absence of fear but the determination to grow despite it.

Not far from the tulip, the **Orchid of Empowerment** blooms with an exotic beauty that captivates all who see it. Its intricate patterns and vibrant hues represent the power of belief in oneself. The orchid reminds the garden that empowerment comes from within and that believing in one's abilities can lead to extraordinary achievements.

Scattered throughout the garden, the **Marigolds of Joy** dance in the sunlight, their golden petals reflecting happiness and content-ment. These flowers, always cheerful and bright, symbolize joy from appreciating life's simple pleasures. The marigolds are the garden's laughter, spreading cheer and positivity to every corner.

In the garden's corners, clusters of **Violets of Kindness** thrive, their soft purple blossoms exuding a gentle beauty. The violets repre-sent the quiet, unassuming nature of kindness, which, though often small and understated, has the power to transform the world around it. Their sweet fragrance fills the garden, reminding every flower that kindness, in its simplicity, is the glue that holds the community together.

You decide that when the rain comes, you will sit on the bench in the heart of your garden, feel the raindrops fall on your body, and be thankful, knowing that the rain is nourishing your flowers. They will grow bigger, stronger, and better. If a destructive storm comes with strong winds and flooding, and leaves behind damage to your garden, you will go to your chest, find the seeds you need, plant them in the empty spots left behind by the storm, and then watch them grow beautiful and even stronger.

You remind yourself that life won't get any easier. You commit to choosing action over inaction. Most importantly, you will tend to your garden and be prepared for any type of weather.

You look up as the sun dips below the horizon, casting a golden glow over the garden; all the flowers stand together, a magnificent mosaic of emotions. Each bloom contributes its unique color, fragrance, and energy, harmonious and balanced.

The garden is a living testament to the power of positive emotions. It is a reminder that when these emotions bloom together in the garden of your heart, they create a life full of love, resilience, and limitless possibilities.

Share your seeds of love and kindness with others. Each seed, no matter how small, has the potential to grow into something beautiful, creating a ripple effect of warmth and compassion that blossoms in the hearts of those it touches.

You take a deep breath and feel an overwhelming amount of gratitude, realizing this is your life. You now know that when you're under pressure, in darkness, pressed, or crushed, you're in a transformation stage, and you will embrace, enjoy, and flourish.

The Journey Inward—
Identify and Uncover the
Emotional Blocks

What are the emotional blocks that prevent you from living the life you desire? These blocks are rooted in unconscious beliefs—stories we've told ourselves for so long that we believe them to be true. "I'm not good enough." "I don't deserve happiness." "I have to put others first." These beliefs are like chains that keep us bound until we recognize and release them.

Your Guide to Freedom and Happiness

Recovering from personal challenges, struggles, and trauma is a journey that requires intention, patience, and self-compassion. This guide provides actionable steps to help you find happiness and reclaim the joy of life.

Imagine a life where the emotional wounds of your past no longer hold you back—a life where you are free to move forward without the weight of old pain dragging you down. The healing process is not just about understanding your pain; it's about actively working to release it and clear the space in your heart and mind for new growth and joy.

The first three steps are of the utmost importance to start your healing journey. This is where you get to the root cause, expose the emotion, release the event and the emotion attached to it, and forgive yourself and any cocreator of the pain you have experienced. You can pick the actionable steps that work best for you in any of the following eight steps.

Step 1: Identifying Your Emotional Blocks

Actionable Steps:

1. Self-reflection

Sit quietly with yourself, free from distractions, and tune into your thoughts and feelings. Notice any recurring patterns or themes that come up—feelings of inadequacy, fear of failure, the need for approval. These clues point to underlying beliefs that may be blocking your path. Ask yourself the tough questions: *What do I believe about myself? Why do I believe this as truth? Where did these beliefs come from? Are they really true?*

Go to the deepest level of the core emotion. The eight basic emotions are joy, trust, fear, surprise, sadness, anticipation, anger, and disgust. If you are feeling fear, what exactly are you feeling? Fear that your friends will think you are lazy, stupid, etc.? Naming your feelings reduces their power over you and, in most cases, will help you identify the root cause of why you feel as you do.

2. Identify patterns

Look at the areas where you feel stuck or dissatisfied. What beliefs might be contributing to these patterns?

3. Journaling

When you find yourself reacting to a trigger, feeling overwhelmed, or overthinking, start writing anything that comes to your mind. You can then look back days later with a clear mind and better understand your emotions and where they come from.

Step 2: Challenging and Releasing Your Blocks

Once you've identified your emotional blocks and their source, the next step is to challenge and release them. Make sure to identify and release the emotion that is attached to the block.

Actionable Steps:

1. Question their validity

Ask yourself: Is this belief really true, or is it just a story I've been telling myself? What evidence do I have to support or refute this belief?

By gathering evidence against your block, you begin to weaken its hold on you.

2. Rewrite the narrative

Once you've challenged a belief, replace it with a new, more empowering one. For instance, instead of "I'm not good enough," you might tell yourself, "I am capable and deserving of success." Repeat this new belief to yourself regularly, especially in moments when the old belief threatens to resurface. Over time, this new belief will take root, and the old block will begin to dissolve.

3. Take responsibility

Take an honest look at the experience and be truthful with yourself about what you could have done differently. If you place all the blame on another person and don't take responsibility for your own actions, you give away your power and control.

4. Visualization

Take a few moments each day to close your eyes and imagine yourself living in alignment with your new belief. Visualize yourself feeling confident, successful, and at peace.

5. Affirmations

Write down your new belief on a piece of paper and place it somewhere you'll see every day—on your bathroom mirror, your computer screen, or your bedside table. Repeat this affirmation to yourself throughout the day, especially in moments of doubt or fear. Repetition will help to reinforce the new belief in your unconscious mind.

6. Journaling

Take time each day to write about your experiences, thoughts, and feelings as you work to release your unconscious beliefs. Journaling allows you to process your emotions, gain insights into your beliefs, and track your progress over time.

Step 3: Forgiveness

True forgiveness is not about absolving others of their wrongs; it's about freeing yourself from the prison of resentment and anger. You must forgive yourself and anyone else involved in the pain you experienced.

Actionable Steps:

1. Write a letter to the person who hurt you

In this letter, express your feelings honestly and openly—what they did, how it affected you, and the pain it caused. Then, as you conclude the letter, make the conscious decision to forgive. You don't have to send the letter; the act of writing it is for your own healing. Once you've written the letter, you can choose to keep it, burn it, or bury it—whatever feels right to symbolize the release of the pain.

2. Forgive yourself

A powerful practice for self-forgiveness is to write down all the things you feel guilty or ashamed about—everything you've been holding against yourself. Then, one by one, consciously release them. Acknowledge the circumstances, understand the context, and then let go of the judgment. As you go through this process, remind yourself that you are human, and that forgiveness is a vital part of your healing journey.

Step 4. Commit to Self-compassion

Practicing self-compassion allows you to accept yourself fully, scars and all.

Actionable Steps:

1. Daily affirmations

Start each day with affirmations that remind you of your worth. Simple phrases like "I am enough," "I am worthy of love and respect," or "I am healing, and it's okay to take my time" help to reprogram your subconscious.

2. Self-compassion journal

After journaling your trauma, write a letter to yourself from the perspective of a loving friend. Similar to chapter six, when you look at your reflection in the mirror, offer yourself the kindness and understanding you would a friend or someone you love.

3. Replace negative self-talk

Notice when you criticize yourself. Acknowledge your thoughts and gently reframe them. For example, if you think, *I should be over this by now,* replace it with, "Healing takes time, and I am doing my best."

Step 5. Establish Boundaries

Setting boundaries will help protect your emotional and mental health and give you control over what you allow into your life.

Actionable Steps:

1. Identify your needs

Reflect on what makes you feel drained, hurt, or unsafe. Write down a list of things you no longer want to tolerate.

2. Communicate clearly

Practice saying no to situations or people who trigger negative emotions or cause you to feel stressed or fearful. Use firm yet respectful language: "I need some space right now," or "I'm not comfortable with this."

3. Reinforce your boundaries

Boundaries are only effective if they're maintained. Hold firm to your decisions, even if others push back. It's okay to prioritize your well-being. By maintaining your boundaries, you control what you choose to allow in your life.

Step 6. Reclaim Your Identity

Emotional pain and trauma can overshadow who we are at our core. Start living the life you want to live. Reconnecting with your true self allows you to regain control of who you are and gives you a sense of purpose.

Actionable Steps:

1. Reconnect with old passions

Think about hobbies or activities you love to do. Dedicate time each week to your personal interests, whether it's music, art, or spending time in nature.

2. Explore new interests

When you turn pain into power, it is an opportunity to change your perspective on life. Use this as an opportunity to explore new passions. Try a class, volunteer, or learn a skill you've always wanted to learn but never did.

Step 7. Build Resilience Through Mindfulness

Mindfulness helps you stay present and calm in the face of over-whelming emotions, allowing you to process your painful events and emotions without being consumed by them.

Actionable Steps:

1. Practice daily meditation

Set aside a minimum of five to ten minutes each day to meditate. Focus on your breath, noticing any sensations in your body without judgment. This helps center your mind and will bring you a sense of tranquility. I have found that meditating in the morning adds value to the whole day.

2. Mindful movement

Engage in gentle activities like yoga, walking, or stretching to re-connect with your body and release tension stored in your muscles.

3. Reflect on your progress

At the end of each week, reflect on your progress. What victories, big or small, have you achieved? Celebrate them. I do this by jour-naling, but you can take a moment to reflect if you prefer.

Step 8. Personal Growth

The primary goal is not just to survive but to thrive. By turning your pain into purpose and wounds into wisdom, you reap the benefits.

Actionable Steps:

1. Recognize your strength

Write down the ways in which your life experience has made you stronger. What lessons have you learned? How have you grown?

2. Give back

Find ways to use your experience to help others. Whether it's through volunteering, mentorship, or advocacy, turning your trauma into a force for good can be incredibly empowering.

The Journey Continues

As you reach the end of this book, you will find that the tools, insights, and practices you've learned here are the foundation for a lifetime of growth, healing, and self-discovery. Continue to build on this foundation, and trust that you have everything you need to create a life of purpose, joy, and fulfillment.

Remember, you are the author of your story, and the future is yours to write. Embrace the journey, cherish the process, and never stop growing. The best is yet to come.

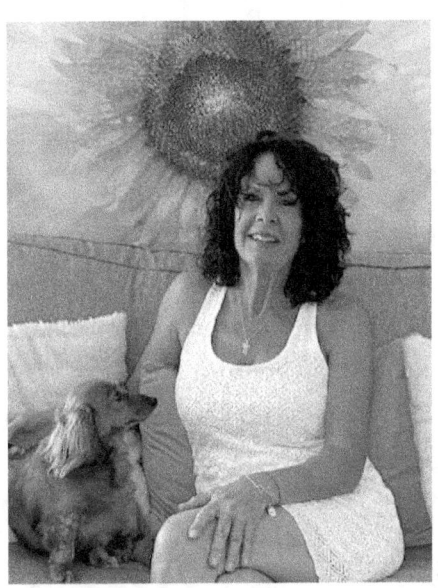

About the Author

Pamela Starusta is a life insurance professional, writer, and advocate for personal growth and healing. Born and raised in Connecticut and now residing in the Tampa Bay area, Pamela has spent her life helping others secure their futures while navigating her own journey through profound personal difficulties. Her experiences have fueled her passion for resilience, emotional wellness, and the strength it takes to rebuild after life's challenges.

Through her career, Pamela has empowered countless families to protect their loved ones, but her true calling extends beyond financial security. She has dedicated herself to exploring the emotional and psychological tools necessary for overcoming life's toughest moments. In *Treasure*, Pamela shares the deeply personal lessons she's learned along the way, offering readers practical advice and inspiration to uncover the gifts hidden in their struggles.

Pamela's mission is to inspire others to embrace their inner strength and transform their pain into purpose. Her insights are rooted in her own recovery and growth, making her guidance heartfelt, relatable, and impactful.

When she's not working or writing, Pamela enjoys traveling, spending time outdoors, and enjoying the power of music. She treasures moments with friends and her beloved mini-dachshund, Violet. Pamela is especially grateful for the unwavering love of her two sons and her family, who have been a constant source of strength and support in her life.

Thank you for joining me on this journey of healing and self-discovery. Your support means everything.

If Treasure resonated with you, please consider leaving a review—it helps spread the message of healing and resilience to others seeking hope and transformation.

Your words have the power to inspire, and I am deeply grateful for your part in sharing this story.

To continue the conversation with Pamela and for additional FREE resources for healing, visit www.PamelaStarusta.com

www.ingramcontent.com/pod-product-compliance
Lightning Source LLC
Chambersburg PA
CBHW070448130626

46553CB00006B/2304